Table of Contents

Nonsustained Ventricular Tachycardia (NSVT) - Outlook and More

Understanding Non-Sustained Ventricular Tachycardia (NSVT)

Nonsustained Ventricular Tachycardia (NSVT) - Outlook and More

1. Introduction to Nonsustained Ventricular Tachycardia (NSVT)

The 1994 American College of Cardiology/American Heart Association guidelines describe a class IIB recommendation for the adjunctive use of an electrophysiologic study (EPS) when a patient presents with a low ejection fraction and NSVT and does not demonstrate a controlled response to exercise testing. Other descriptions in this report suggest an association with progression to sustained VT and provide a class IIB recommendation (if they are inducible) for an ICD in patients with an EF<40% with NSVT caused by prior MI. There is no information in this report to suggest treatment options or description for low ejection fraction and negative exercise testing with NSVT.

The prevalence of NSVT varies in different heart diseases. In a relatively young and healthy population of firefighters who underwent serial annual follow-up exams and robust stress tests for over 10 years, NSVT is a frequent finding of a normal physiological response and is also more common among black and obese men. Frequent NSVT in these populations is an incidental observation and is a risk marker for advanced age, smoking, and chronic hypertension and unrelated to coronary artery disease. Independent of age, the prevalence of NSVT is higher in men, decreasing with age, and NSVTs become almost non-detectable among persons in the higher age-groups. Interestingly, the prevalence of NSVT as a risk marker for persons <40 years of age is "expectedly" higher in black subjects compared with white subjects. There is no significant correlation between exercise-induced atrial or atrioventricular nodal response and the occurrence of NSVT. In diseased populations, the prevalence of NSVT is more common in individuals with a history of myocardial infarction, heart failure, coronary revascularization (all types), various structural heart diseases, and primary electrical diseases including inherited and inflammatory conditions.

Nonsustained ventricular tachycardia (NSVT) is defined by the occurrence of a relatively short run or sequence of irregular heartbeats from the ventricle of more than 3 beats, but terminating spontaneously within 30 seconds, without any hemodynamic compromise. Pathophysiologically, NSVT can be explained by various mechanisms and may be accompanied by occult or clinically significant cardiac structural or electrophysiological abnormalities.

2. Epidemiology and Prevalence

In an early study from Rochester, Minnesota, a high prevalence of approximately 5% amongst individuals was noted though no significant distinction in age (20 to 94) or sex was found. In a study of clinically healthy middle-aged individuals with no known heart disease residing in Olmsted County, Minnesota, the 10-year cumulative incidence rate of symptomatic NSVT was 0.7%, comprising of 16.6% with idiopathic, 33.3% with borderline, and 50% with overt heart disease. In Japan, NSVT were found to be prevalent in 4, 2, and 1% according to sex among 22,209 subjects. Here, the prevalence of NSVT increased with age in both sexes. It was more common in men than women over the age of 50 but showed no sex differences between 20 and 49 years.

The prevalence of NSVT in the general population is largely unknown. This is in part because in most individuals, isolated NSVTs go unnoticed and remain asymptomatic. The incidence rate of isolated NSVT in the presence of underlying heart disease is approximately 14-15 cases per 100,000 person-years, whereas in the absence of structural heart disease, isolated NSVTs can be recorded in around 2-3 cases per 100,000. A greater proportion of patients with symptomatic heart failure are found to have NSVT than asymptomatic individuals (33% vs. 10-13%), and NSVT becomes more common with advancing age in patients without heart failure. The prevalence of NSVT increases with age and is more common in men than in women.

There was no significant difference found between men and women for faster heart rates; however, women have been found to have significantly slower heart rates for all coupling intervals compared to men, and this is said to be a potential explanation for the observed higher prevalence of NSVT in men. Overall, NSVT is frequently detected with wide variability in prevalence rates reported due to differences in definition, duration, age, sex, region, and setting.

2.1. Global Incidence Rates

Results/Significance. The global incidence of NSVT, after excluding frequent premature ventricular complexes, is estimated to occur between 4.6% and 12.3% of the antithrombotic heart failure cohort. Female and white patients with somewhat controlled rates of heart disease and non-IHD have slightly higher risks of NSVT. The range of NSVT may be expected to decrease with higher doses of atenolol (5 lower motivation to continue). The summary incidence of NSVT is 1.8% (5 of 7) after atenolol washout and increases to 12.3% (9 of 73) in 6 weeks (upper limit of 95% CI 21.3%) in part because doctors focused on the WHI, TPT, and SOF to select patients at somewhat higher risk of adverse events.

Background. A basic area is important to serve as a reference for the frequency of occurrence of nonsustained ventricular tachycardia (NSVT). This will partially address the epidemiology of the short-lasting arrhythmia. Representative populations in terms of diseases and disorders were used to study whether the incidence rate would be on the preventative side of the equation. This information is important if sizable samples of heart patients are to be assessed with longer monitoring.

2.2. Age and Gender Distribution

Some reports have managed to identify warning signs from an existing NSVT. Family background suggesting a weird illness is often recognized as a possibility but seems very strange. Conn and Colco reported chances of sudden demise about 7 in 510 uninhibited NSVT survivors, respectively. A single review reported severe harm or unforeseen demise as numerous incidents in 300 RATE participants of 72, generally associated with hypertrophy undetectable with only electrocardiograms, myocardial infarction, or just hyperactive NSVT at the time of inspection. On the other hand, 9, three of the 23 people in the experience (13%) were damaged in this collective in the same general population. Atrial fibrillation and congestive failure are both considered primary illnesses. MaCGUIRE noted on the left ventricular systolic function in 80 patients and noted short tachycardia characters inserted into the unusual NSAID expected in many individuals on weekdays. These experience members could assume that mesoses of resting and activity could not have been physical damage through antiarrhythmic medication. Harari found that 17 of the 87 members showed astonishing physical injury on experienced detervdual, current CTC electrocardiograms to have the minimum left-mead systolic constitutional performance claimed in clinical management. Assume that the previously referenced studies do not serve to resolve this danger. Presumably, for SKISTON included in the survey, anterior ST-T amendment finals set a detailed bladder signal in a minicomputer version tagged root for catheterization for 6.5 sessions of experience, that hardly determines that the two notice in the bodies of 22 agents should be probable, HIV or 29% in six, according to procedures not connected with physical discomfort.

Age and gender distribution: Normally, people older than 35 are mostly suffering, and triggers seem to stay stable throughout age. The majority of doctors are optimistic in their prediction of children's symptoms, so the existence of symptoms in children irritates everyone. On the other hand, one and a half people have agreed that those who have invalid drugs have been worried in the long term. After 198 employees conducted a fast test to calculate the frequency on newly established SVT patients in the universal mid-forty, professionals showed no fact that necessity can predict an attack.

Nonsustained ventricular tachycardia is a serious but under-investigated condition. But which subpopulations are more affected than others? Preliminary key elements or old risk factors are mostly being used to connect to the foundation. There are numerous warnings in medical practice that have allowed offbeat effects in several respects to pursue further analysis.

3. Pathophysiology of NSVT

The most common mechanisms underlying NSVT in the ATHENA registry were focal (58.9%), followed by reentry (41.1%). Reentry is the underlying arrhythmogenesis of NSVT in several acquired and inherited conditions. Slowly conducting or unidirectional block in ischemia facilitates the reentry. Also, pericardial fat (especially in obese patients), Purkinje, or reconnecting fibers may play a role, the latter with late potential on the ECG. Automaticity is associated with voltage gradients in ischemic myocardium responsible for premature beats. The pathophysiology of triggered activity mostly results from an increase in cytoplasmic free Ca+2 concentration secondary to reduced Ca-ATPase, underactivity of SR Ca2+ ATPase, Na+/Ca+2 exchange, and stress or exercise.

Nonsustained ventricular tachycardia (NSVT) is observed in approximately 20% to 50% of patients during 24-hour ambulatory electrocardiography (ECG). Various mechanisms participate in the genesis of NSVT, including reentrant mechanisms, triggered and automatic activity, bradycardia-dependent and alteration of cardiac autonomic function, which can be associated in some instances. Their studies showed that despite a higher occurrence of PVCs and NSVTs in non-ischemic patients, NSVT was idiopathic in only 25%. The underlying pathophysiology of NSVT is quite complex and dependent on the underlying etiology as well as specific individual factors. This partially explains the variable clinical scenarios observed in these patients. The three principal mechanisms of arrhythmogenesis in NSVT include reentry, automaticity, and triggered activity.

3.1. Electrophysiological Mechanisms

Arrhythmias are developed in heart disease. The cells of the myocardium are subjected to electrical and morphological changes that favor the occurrence of circulating wavefronts of electrical activity. These wavefronts pass along abnormal excitable tissue pathways in the heart and are unable to continue re-entering the same tissue regions. One form of arrhythmia is called nonsustained ventricular tachycardia (NSVT). During NSVT, the heart rate is suddenly much faster than the normal 60 to 100 beats per minute, but the duration of the arrhythmia is limited to 100-120 beats. It is a topic of clinical interest as it is associated with an increased risk of major adverse outcomes. The mechanisms responsible for NSVT are still poorly understood. It is generally thought to involve an important part of functional tissue (i.e., tissue that is likely to recover and therefore become excitable over time) that re-enters a certain number of millimeters of electrically inactive heart tissue and continues to recover normally until it re-enters the initiating region.

Abstract: Nonsustained ventricular tachycardia (NSVT) arises from abnormal electrical activity in the heart and is associated with an increased risk of major adverse outcomes. Although the electrophysiological mechanisms that lead to NSVT remain incompletely understood, there is evidence that activation of the sympathetic nervous system, often in response to physical or emotional stress, elicits cardiac electrical changes that favor reentrant activities, thereby making NSVT more likely. In experimental models of heart disease, NSVT can also occur because of premature ventricular action potentials that lead to several cycles of early-afterdepolarization-mediated triggered activity; however, the role of this mechanism in patients remains to be demonstrated. Current treatments for NSVT have antiarrhythmic actions that are not cardio-specific. Ongoing studies are working to develop therapies that have a very specific action to terminate reentrant activities in patients.

3.2. Underlying Cardiac Conditions

Electrical and structural remodeling occurs in the myocardium in the course of hypertension as well, especially in the presence of LV hypertrophy, myocardial fibrotic scar tissue mass, which facilitates repolarization anomalies and the occurrence of arrhythmias. This is the basis for the appearance of arrhythmias caused by drug intoxications, genetic disorders, and physical, chemical influences. In heredodegenerative diseases and in cases accompanied by functional changes in the cell organelles (reticulosarcoma, cardiomyopathies, cardiac amyloidosis), the described complications of calcium handling can also be found. Furthermore, different viruses (coxsackie, echovirus, adenovirus, cytomegalovirus), Lyme-borrelia, diarrhea-pandemic or other myocarditis pathogens can, in addition to myocarditis, induce inflammatory signals, increasing the risk of malignant arrhythmias.

Chronic heart diseases, such as coronary heart disease, myocardial infarction, ventricular hypertrophy, myocarditis, or hydropericarditis, increase the development of arrhythmias through an increased dispersion of ventricular repolarization. In these cases, mitochondriosis and cytoplasmic calcinosis can be formed, the accumulated Ca+ reaches the T tubules, or alters calcium ATPase function in the myocardial cells. Practically, slow arrhythmias can be observed in these cases, while low blood flow facilitates ischemia. The reason for the increased potential of pathological focus development pertains to altered ventricular myocardial blood supply, electrolyte metabolism, and residence time, its pathological heterogeneity.

4. Clinical Manifestations

NSVT can be classified based on onset: it can occur in people without underlying heart disease (usually in patients using agents that enhance sympathetic activity called positive inotropic or vasodilator drugs) and those with cardiac disease. The second type usually appears during a 24-hour cardiac monitoring test after heart attack, or in individuals with minimal coronary artery disease before missing the six to eighteen months following a heart attack, ventricular hypertrophy or pre-excitation syndrome. A standard 12-channel ECG, cardiac imaging and testing, tilt-table testing, as well as chest X-ray procedures can identify potential underlying causes. If the arrhythmia becomes sustained and/or resistant to treatment, more advanced methods such as electrophysiological catheterization and endocardial or epicardial ablation are considered.

Nonsustained ventricular tachycardia (NSVT) is defined as a rapid rhythm originating from the ventricles (structures below the atria in the heart) with varying heart acceleration, which usually lasts for between three and 30 beats. NSVT can be classified based on its QRS duration: polymorphic (<120 msec); more frequently occurring monomorphic that degenerates into polymorphic; and monomorphic, which originates in the right or left ventricle and spreads to either side, causing a wide (≥120 msec) and bizarre QRS complex prior to more accelerating heart contractions. The most common causes of NSVT are ischemic heart disease and structural heart disease, but other conditions such as electrolyte imbalances, iatrogenic induction, neoplasms, infections, poisons, etc., can indirectly affect the heart, resulting in this tachycardia. While some individuals remain symptom-free, presenting only an altered resting ECG, others evidence palpitations, chest pain, dyspnea, presyncope and syncope due to the brief decrease in blood flow.

4.1. Symptoms and Presentation

In summary, the majority are asymptomatic, and emergency therapy should focus on the underlying disorder in symptom alleviating the comparative portion of patients. Fear or anxiety might be a similar negative factor in people with palpitations due to NSVT. A small number of patients do value recognition on the basis of NSVT detection or benefit from specific chest pain avoidance protocols.

Clinicians should have a low threshold for discussing symptoms of patients with NSVT and making relevant assessments, particularly in those identified to be at high risk of complications. A detailed assessment, including 12-lead ECG, 24-h ECG holter, and discussion with a heart rhythm specialist to determine the mechanism of arrhythmia and associated risk factors, may help alleviate concerns and enable the best possible care for patients.

According to a population-based arrhythmia study, those who reported dizziness or fainting had a higher ventricular premature beat counts and runs of nonsustained ventricular tachycardia (NSVT), and those with syncope, in particular, presented with more frequent ventricular ectopic beats. Chest pain and anxiety have been reported as other potential symptoms of NSVT, although these are more likely to be due to the underlying pathology, e.g., pre-existing coronary artery disease or stress, rather than due to the short bursts of rapid arrhythmia per se.

Regardless of the underlying mechanism of NSVT, the likelihood of patients presenting with symptoms during tachycardia episodes, such as palpitations, dizziness, or syncope, appears to be low. However, in those who have structural heart disease (SHD), the symptoms are likely to be associated with a higher burden of NSVT, suggesting that the extent of ventricular arrhythmia might determine the clinical presentation.

4.2. Diagnostic Evaluation

The LVEF and serum biomarkers should be measured early in the index event, and the remaining tests should be scheduled based on the clinical stability, available diagnostic facilities, type of event (NSVT onset), outpatient or in-patient pathways. A sorbitol positron emission tomography scan, early coronary angiographic assessment or ergonovine testing if suspicion or exclusion criterion for coronary artery disease should be considered if arranged by an advanced heart team. It is also important and relevant to advise the patient to avoid activities and behaviors that trigger or precipitate the onset of NSVT, such as alcohol, nicotine, caffeine, sleep deprivation, and substances like cocaine and other stimulants.

The diagnostic procedure can be classified in initial evaluation of diagnostic suspicion, evaluation of extent and diagnostic classification, and risk stratification and risk stratification electric evaluation. The initial evaluation should be based on the clinical symptoms obtained from the patient and other supplementary studied heart disease, medication such as the existence of drugs that support the long QT, and personal or family history of sudden cardiac death. The radioplethysmographic ECG with V1-V2 rhythm strips analysis may aid diagnosis by capturing the NSVT. Also, a resting ECG is suitable to assure classification on the QRS, which is associated with structural heart disease and risk stratification. However, most individuals should proceed to additional testing in- or outpatient.

The diagnosis of NSVT must be suspected in any individual with the clinical history described before who presents with palpitations, a clear awareness of 'heart skipping beats', or when detected incidentally by LVEF or ambulatory ECG tests (Holter, external/holter). Therefore, a proper clinical history, a resting 12-lead ECG and a LVEF measurement or any of the aforementioned tests are the cornerstone of diagnosis.

5. Risk Stratification in NSVT

Cardiac structural changes and impaired left ventricular function have important values in the risk stratification of patients with NSVT; this explains the important role for an electrophysiology study. Most common scores for risk stratification in patients with structural heart disease range from coronary artery disease to a long-term prognosis assessment, as reported. Patients with hypertrophic cardiomyopathy that suffer from NSVT during Holter monitoring and present one more risk factor for SCD, as identified by the HCM Risk-SCD score, should be considered for an ICD. In coronary heart disease, Holter monitoring is performed to determine the ability to carry on with therapy. An electrophysiology study may be indicated in the case of ischemic cardiomyopathy and a frequent occurrence of NSVT on 24-hour recording. For myotonic dystrophy, the value of an electrophysiology study in risk stratification should be proven. The results of a stress test on determining the need for primary prevention ICD may be different, especially when performed soon after myocardial infarction or revascularization. To date, in patients with a borderline ejection fraction (<35 and >30), more attention should be paid.

Nonsustained ventricular tachycardia (NSVT) is a complex and intriguing arrhythmic phenomenon that involves multiple factors, including cardiac and noncardiac factors, to be solved. The last frontier for the management of patients with NSVT is represented by the definition of the role of electrophysiology study in risk stratification of patients with NSVT; its role is somewhat limited, and workloads on electrophysiology studies need to be defined. Moreover, no specific treatment for NSVT has been described; in fact, not all the patients benefit from ICD therapy. Risk stratification is nonetheless essential; moreover, risk stratification on the basis of NSVT needs to identify patients who may benefit from long-term therapy with an ICD, including the type of NSVT and the underlying disease. To date, NSVT resulting in a diagnosis of "malignant arrhythmia" (ventricular tachycardia) is deeply unknown; it is also crucial to define more objective rhythms that can be stratified by considering repetitive appearances over a longer period.

5.1. Prognostic Indicators

Below are the reported risk indicators of the great majority of the prognostic studies. Some recent studies have not incorporated some of them because they were mainly designed to test the benefit of a prophylactic non-selective, ICD therapy and needed evident significant life-threatening arrhythmias for inclusion in the randomized patients. Moreover, most articles were published more than 15 years ago in small, conflicting and not representative samples, primarily about patients who donated themselves to undergo an EPS.

The clinical significance of NSVT lies in its potential for progression to life-threatening ventricular arrhythmias or occurrence of arrhythmic syncope, which need in turn to be predicted by available diagnostic factors. Some factors or risk markers, which entering into multivariate analyses of primarily selected populations finally could be obtained as independent predictors by most authors, may not always be fully consistent, when results from both all available reports and a more recent paper by Albert et al. are reviewed. It is clinically of interest that no definite proof has been presented yet that electrophysiological testing (EPS) would be very helpful in triggering ICD therapy in a specific high-risk group of patients mainly on the basis of a more efficient prediction of VT events. The clinical value of all prognostic indicators needs ultimately to be judged by the relevance of the respective risk for risk formulation and optimal local management choice in the clinical context of the whole-patient picture and of the real-life conditions, including the advent of ICDs.

5.2. Scoring Systems

In tachyarrhythmia, two different scores address the same issue of atrial fibrillation, chronic heart failure, and hypertension, with the EHRA/HRS score assigned for appropriateness for ICD implantation. The use of scoring systems in NSVT creates an opportunity to formalize the risk assessment and the decision-making progression as well as services necessary to reduce the risk of SCD. Furthermore, it enables the identification of individuals who may need further investigations to determine the exact cause of the NSVT. Even though a scoring system is not applicable for a patient with NSVT right after the 72-hour assessment duration, if symptoms persist or new complaints emerge.

Two structured approaches are available employing a sum of points, where the value expressed as the number of points corresponds to the value's categorical location within the relevant condition. Bigger numbers mean higher risk. The NYHA classification is based mainly on symptoms, despite symptoms being known to be a predictor of outcome as well. The aLQTS score likewise uses the sum of points method and takes into account established risk factors, which is the main difference between the two, as it is a risk prediction model.

5.2. Scoring Systems

With the increasing knowledge about the underlying mechanisms and prognostic and therapeutic implications, a question arises as to how the risk assessment should be performed. One way of doing this is scoring systems, which are not only recommended in preventive cardiology.

6. Management Strategies

Pharmacological Intervention If the primary aim is to manage the symptom load in the form of palpitations, dizziness or syncope, hence the management of refractory or symptomatic NSVT would focus more upon the suppression of ventricular ectopics or tachycardia. Beta-blockers are considered a first-line option in the medical management of patients with NSVT, irrespective of the underlying cause. If they are insufficient or not preferred, calcium-channel blockers and class I antiarrhythmic drugs can also be considered. In accordance with the current guidelines, amiodarone is not currently recommended as first-line pharmacological therapy in patients with heart failure and a reduced ejection fraction, NSVT and myocardial infarction. Furthermore, amiodarone use for the primary prevention of sudden cardiac death is associated with the overall increase in mortality. Amiodarone due to its side effect profile including pulmonary fibrosis, thyroid, and hepatic toxicity, corneal micro-deposits, qt-prolongation and squamous cell carcinoma, as well as higher dose of usage, and prolonged exposure to the drug cause more adverse reactions in Asians and is generally avoided worldwide. Hence it is always considered and used cautiously accompanied with periodic monitoring.

Management The evaluation of NSVT is principally focused on defining the clinical significance or the substrate that can lead to the development of ventricular tachyarrhythmia in the future. Management of NSVT is largely divided into pharmacological therapy and catheter ablation. At present, there are no pharmacological options found to be associated with mortality benefit. However, suppression of NSVT might be considered in cases of underlying ventricular dysfunction and heart failure symptoms. Catheter ablation of individuals with structural heart disease can be performed both in the form of radiofrequency and cryoablation of rapidly firing focal triggers, termed idiopathic NSVT, or the underlying reentry substrate guided by diagnostic electrophysiological mapping. Discussion regarding the invasive management of VT would require a separate article altogether.

6.1. Pharmacological Interventions

Although the use of antiarrhythmic drugs is associated with side effects and there is a need for pharmacologic management in all types of tachyarrhythmias originated from the ventricle, continuous exposure to these drugs leads to pharmacologic-induced, structural ventricle-myocardial injuries when parasympathetic and sympathetic systems regulate the operation of the heartbeats through cardiac adrenergic receptors. Even when the drug is stopped, some changes in the expression of cardiac adrenergic receptor and the reabsorption system slow down, thereby increasing the rate of convert manganese. The expressions of adrenergic and muscarinic receptors in Sino-Atrial node varies depending on the resting and minimal contractile heart rates. Additionally, taking any antiarrhythmic drug is known to be an independent risk factor for a minor or major hospital admission during first 6 months and post-discharge.

Antiarrhythmic drugs are used to manage nonsustained ventricular tachycardia (NSVT), suppressing arrhythmias effectively through different pathways. As for NSVT, however, most of the drugs used were only indicated for high-risk groups who were also suffering from myocardial infarction or dilated cardiac myopathy. Given the fact that the prognosis of NSVT derived from different sites is equivocal but might be better than expected, most drugs and dosage energy would be recommended based on the Consensus Report for the Management of Ventricular Arrhythmias Except Sudden Cardiac Death released by the

American College of Cardiology (ACC), the American Heart Association (AHA), and the European Society of Cardiology (ESC) in 1985. This report underlines no fixed standardized treatments were available for patients, citing administration with or without drugs during acute management. When choosing the medications that suppress ventricular tachycardia caused by NSVT, it is important to assess the estimated cause of arrhythmia, in addition to the mechanism of arrhythmia. The most common cause of ventricular tachycardia of NSVT is idiopathic, but arrhythmias developed from organic heart disease may be related to a worse prognosis and co-existing arrhythmias such as atrial fibrillation or flutter.

6.2. Catheter Ablation

NSVT and idiopathic ventricular arrhythmias have a good outcome and therefore are an attractive object for testing efficacy and safety of new ablation tools. Although data are much less in number compared to all supraventricular tachycardias, a classification considering the known etiology of the arrhythmia can still be done to guide clinical management. Successful elimination of NSVT is able to stabilize the myocardial substrate and has been shown to prevent additional life-threatening ventricular arrhythmias and sudden cardiac death in ischemic heart disease with left ventricular dysfunction, known arrhythmic right ventricular cardiomyopathy, catecholaminergic polymorphic ventricular tachycardia, Brugada syndrome, and early repolarization syndrome. Clinicians involved in the management of individuals with NSVT should be familiar with the potential contemporary procedural intervention for NSVT as catheter ablation has been firmly established.

Outcomes of catheter ablation according to NSVT underlying disease:

Catheter ablation aims to directly interrupt the underlying pathophysiological substrate or break the arrhythmia cycle by targeting reentry circuits. In ventricular tachycardias and hence in most cases of NSVT, the focus is to control the underlying disease. Therefore, ablation procedures are only recommended in high-risk conditions with a high likelihood to deteriorate to symptoms or to ventricular fibrillation and sudden cardiac death or distinct symptomatic tachycardias.

Management approach to catheter ablation, principles, and outcomes for NSVT:

7. Outcomes and Prognosis

In rare cases of NSVT in patients with previously diagnosed coronary artery disease, previous myocardial infarction, nonischemic cardiomyopathies, and CHF/LV dysfunction and recently discovered to have NSVT, based on meta-analyses, we expect a sudden death risk of about 7% to 9% over a 2 to 3 year period. Potential complications are associated with further losses of functioning or systems, development of secondary paroxysmal and fatal arrhythmias following recurrence chromic LV systolic dysfunction in ARIC cohort 20 plus year observed a mortality rate of 17% of the subjects. LV Systolic Dysfunction was observed in half of individuals with NSVT in the Harvard cohort study with fatal arrhythmias accounting for similar rates of morbidity which were observed in NSVT with exercise stress testing. LV dilatation and dysfunction have been infrequently observed evolve from NSVT.

One of the most common questions we get as clinicians is, "What is the prognosis associated with nonsustained ventricular tachycardia (NSVT)?" In the setting of a structurally normal heart and no historical features of syncope, generally, the prognosis and outcomes are excellent based on long-term follow-up studies. That being said, it's also important to understand that, even in a structurally normal heart, nonsustained ventricular tachycardia (NSVT) can be present to some extent immediately prior to sudden cardiac death or a malignant arrhythmic event. This being the case, some fraction of relatively rare circumstances of NSVT can certainly lead to a poor outcome.

7.1. Long-Term Follow-Up Studies

Long-term follow-up studies on individuals with NSVT are important, reminding us that a significant number continue to be free from potentially lethal ventricular arrhythmias or sudden death over time. With this study's long follow-up, it can accurately be said that the majority of individuals will not have malignant ventricular arrhythmias over time. Certain individuals are, however, at risk of sudden death and a thorough evaluation is necessary. When investigating the risk of sudden death, we found that systolic dysfunction was the solitary independent predictor. Even though many individuals had totally normal echocardiograms or other triggers for ventricular arrhythmias according to the scientific literature, no or minute structural heart disease could not alone ascertain a benign outcome. Only a device intervention may possibly raise prolonged existence, as these patients have a better outcome post device implantation. There is no significant dissimilarity in outcome between older and younger individuals. The absence of symptoms likewise is not of prognostic price in individuals with NSVT, no matter what their age.

The prognostic value of nonsustained ventricular tachycardia (NSVT) is often discussed in conjunction with other predictors of sudden cardiac death. While short-term or intermediate follow-up is often performed in primary prevention intervention, long-term follow-up data adds substantial support when predicting outcome. Studies with extended follow-up solely focusing on individuals with

NSVT have revealed that most individuals remain stable over time, and that it seems that the need for device therapy is relatively low. This section will delve into the results from these studies, discussing how ventricular arrhythmias fare in the long run and offering a non-exhaustive list of different variables employed to evaluate the association of NSVT with outcome in extended follow-up studies. Clinicians can use the following information to inform both prognosis and clinical management at first presentation of NSVT.

7.2. Complications and Mortality Rates

There is a paucity of data available detailing exact mortality rates due to nonsustained ventricular tachycardia. Indeed, the multicenter trial that was conducted with patients stratified for primary and secondary prevention of sudden death does comment on mortality due to arrhythmic death (exacerbation of nonsustained ventricular arrhythmias to sustained rhythm) following nonsustained ventricular tachycardia in patients implanted with ICDs, but does not cite overall crude mortality rates specifically resulting from NSVT. Despite tried and tested risk assessment tools, appropriate patient selection (in terms of the qualification of congestive heart failure, myocardial infarction and durability of the VT, among other factors) will remain the most important aspect in establishing who and when individuals might progress to developing life-threatening ventricular arrhythmia. It must be acknowledged that these tools are far from perfect when it comes to their predictive capabilities.

Nonsustained ventricular tachycardia (NSVT) is a typically benign condition in otherwise healthy individuals. However, understanding adverse consequences, if any, as well as mortality resulting from it, is important. By understanding complications and mortality rates, a better idea of acute and long-term prognosis can be established, while providing this information accurately to patients can drive more valid informed consent. Moreover, being able to effectively zero in on the risk profile of a patient group can significantly enhance the ability to provide nuanced and therefore more targeted treatment as well as lifestyle and self-care advice. Complications that may occur as a result of NSVT include the risk of ventricular fibrillation (VF) or sudden cardiac death (SCD), resulting either from ongoing or faster tachycardia or reentry. More commonly, progression of disease to a clinical level of VT (including sustained VT and electrical storm), ICD interventions, anxiety, and poor patient quality of life have all been described.

8. Future Directions in NSVT Research

The cardiac autonomic nervous system (ANS) likely participates in NSVT originating in the normal heart. While we currently have the means to treat the electrical consequence, NSVT, our understanding of the cellular processes leading to hemangioma progression to BAVB are limited. However, image-derived indices of electromechanical coupling, such as integrating cardiomechanical coupling efficiency and the non-compensated ventricular workload that impact ventriculo-ventricular function, may provide insight and additional evaluation tools in the overall treatment approach. Research is ongoing to further refine our understanding of this subset of patients.

The importance of many episodes of nonsustained ventricular tachycardia (NSVT) continues to be debated. While we still do not have an easy, non-invasive method to reliably diagnose arrhythmic syncope, advances in non-invasive diagnosis such as multi-electrode recordings of body surface potential and electrode arrays for cellular electrophysiology are providing development tools for very precise diagnosis and prognosis. New approaches to the treatment of NSVT in heart disease, both in fair hearts and in hypertrophic cardiomyopathy, are in development. It may be possible to provide definitive therapy for ventricular tachycardia in many patients by targeting the ganglia of the heart rather than the myocardium to suppress NSVT. As imaging improves and informs the locations of the ganglia, while new computer modeling demonstrates how ganglia may be calculating the heart rate and blood pressure, a complete understanding of the cardiac autonomic nervous system could make such therapy routine, translating into improved clinical outcomes.

Future Directions

8.1. Advances in Diagnostic Technologies

Ventricular tachycardia causes the highest death toll among the over-65s in the United States. At least several outcomes are significantly reduced when planning or surveying essential exams for the treatment or exhaustion of tachycardiomyopathy cured by catheters. We've got a phone that can't be done; existing confusion; speculation and absence of sturdy indigenous capabilities leading to generations of leisure activities and facilities. Dividends. To date, pacemakers and CRT tools cannot be activated to safely and efficiently save Atr. Our report capitalizes on a new and quickly upgradable community arrhythmia control process described in the current literature. Developed by the Rome - RED, this is a multi-electrode limited (epidermal skin) white light of a long-term record. Tachyarrhythmias are detected by testing statistical reliability on R-R repeat bronchoscopy using substitute (hidden Markov) models. It has gained quick consent for multimodal care via night clinic and fingertip clinics and causes dyspnea around the heart attack area. The internet node includes real internet cafes stored high file. Furmans includes an edge to segment pathological QPLUS tears. Dynamic ECG evaluation is not limited in time in NSVT testing managing.

Eighty-six years after the first identification of NSVT during cardiac angiography, depending on the hospital, the mean endpoint for survival without SVT births was six months. Eleven percent of UUS participated with SVT due to LVSS at the time of an external defibrillator implant. Memetics studies are suitable for showing prolonged R-R variability in the human population coping with community-gained coronary thromboembolic infarction (valley variability) and identifying beepers before heart failure.

8.2. Innovative Treatment Approaches

The prejudice of NSVT as a benign electrocardiographic entity is vanishing away, as a new finding showcases its independent increased risk of HF hospitalization and sudden cardiac death. Mortality in the reported studies indicates the importance of early interventions in patients with greater NSVT burden to halt the deterioration of the left ventricular function. Emerging evidence points with medications like iglifolin, beta blockers, amiodarone, and nicorandil undergoing trials across the globe for probable efficacy in NSVT patients. If proven, medications like ivabradine, filtering and non-filtering antiarrhythmics, cardiac contractility modulators, and new drugs like chornotrophin, antisense oligonucleotide, and arginine vasopressinase (nanosomodulation) can also jump start for possible treatments in this population in future.

Medications like beta blockers, amiodarone, and verapamil, routinely used for ventricular tachycardia management, are currently under the lens for possible antiarrhythmic activities in NSVT. On the other hand, radiofrequency ablation may join the league for the treatment of frequent NSVT, following the difficulties in the medication therapies. Different studies are currently underway to test the efficacy of radiofrequency ablation in patients with frequent NSVT of different etiologies. Recently, the use of nanosomodulation for ventricular tachycardia has emerged and it will be interesting to investigate in the future whether a shorter version of nanosomodulation treatment is effective for patients with neuromodular bundle ventricular tachycardia.

Understanding Non-Sustained Ventricular Tachycardia (NSVT)

1. Introduction to NSVT

Non-sustained ventricular tachycardia is defined as a rapid, usually regular, ventricular rhythm lasting for a short amount of time when its duration is defined in seconds. It occurs most frequently in individuals with persistent ventricular tachycardia (VT), those with structural heart disease that either are asymptomatic or have symptoms that can be less consistently reproduced. It may also be seen in individuals with other forms of heart disease or inherited conditions. Sustained VT is the most critical arrhythmic manifestation of heart disease, causing fainting, a sudden drop in blood pressure, severe dyspnea, chest pain, and ventricular fibrillation.

The heart's rhythm is usually steady, controlled by electrical signals sent across the heart's chambers. When these signals are disrupted, the heart can begin to beat much faster than it should. This condition is referred to as non-sustained ventricular tachycardia (NSVT) and causes the heart to beat between 100 and 250 times per minute, most often in individuals with a pre-existing heart condition. While NSVT only affects the body for a short time, it can lead to more dangerous heart conditions if left untreated. This paper will touch on key aspects of NSVT and provide further details on its manifestation, when it is diagnosed, the risk factors and associated symptoms, how it is treated, and which long-term prognosis individuals have.

1.1. Definition and Overview

The immediate and accurate definition of NSVT is where three or more consecutive beats occur at a rate faster than 120 beats per minute and are terminated within 30 seconds. Along with this basic definition, some pieces of information are required to better define NSVT in absolute terms. Health professionals need some details such as the regularity and frequency of the beats. The causes of NSVT are wide-ranging, stemming from psychological factors or differing states of pathology within the body. Although this condition is low risk and often goes undiagnosed, NSVT can still indicate the presence of underlying diseases and should be properly managed at the primary healthcare level. It is therefore important to explore the relationship between NSVT and health conditions, as well as the clinical impact of asymptomatic NSVT, in order to better understand what is at stake.

Non-sustained ventricular tachycardia (NSVT) refers to a noticeably rapid heartbeat initiated by an irregular electrical impulse. Although NSVT can last for approximately 30 seconds or longer, it fizzles on its own and does not necessitate medical intervention. NSVT can cause a rapid but regular heartbeat and may arise from the ventricles of the heart. Efficient treatments exist to manage NSVT and, subsequently, eradicate any potential distress. Ventricular tachycardia (VT) is a condition that generates an accelerated heart rate and raises the likelihood of sudden cardiac arrest and other cardiovascular diseases in severe cases.

1.2. Prevalence and Risk Factors

The prevalence and risk factors of NSVT were also poorly understood before the Hamburg City Health Study (HCHS) included the Miniature Electrocardiography in the Home-based IntraVascular Screening (MEHIVIS) study, which collected the data reported in this thesis (see also supplementary Abb.). A better understanding of the prevalence and risk factors of NSVT is needed because of the potential risk of developing sustained ventricular tachycardia, the psychological impact on people who have experienced NSVT (i.e., arrhythmophobia), and to consider preventive measures for the development of NSVT. Atrial fibrillation (AF), long QT-interval duration, and male sex were associated with an increased prevalence of NSVT in the HCHS. In the ARIC study, smoking, history of coronary heart disease, and AF were related to the presence of NSVT. The LURIC study showed an increased risk for NSVT by several CVD risk factors, such as smoking, low HDL-cholesterol, dilated left atrium, history of myocardial infarction, and elevated plasma cardiac troponin I, copeptin, and MR-proANP. Also, although we demonstrated that there was an independent positive association between the length of the QTc interval and the occurrence of NSVT, the association with NSVT disappeared after additional adjustment with presence of cardiovascular risk factors.

2. Symptoms of NSVT

2.1. Palpitations and Chest Discomfort

2.2. Dizziness and Lightheadedness

3. Diagnosis of NSVT

The electrocardiogram (ECG) is the first-line investigation in the assessment of patients with palpitations or anyone perceived to have had a cardiac event, including syncope. The characteristic appearance of NSVT on the ECG (Figure 1) may be diagnostic and reveal the underlying mechanism. When a patient is symptomatic, rhythm interrogation may detect isolated premature ventricular complexes (PVCs); pulse and QRS character are useful in differentiating supraventricular tachycardia with bundle branch block from NSVT.

As NSVT episodes are often asymptomatic and have a self-terminating nature, evidence to support treatment modalities specific for NSVT (irrespective of triggering factors) is limited. Consequently, accurate identification of NSVT is key and would typically involve further investigations should it be suspected. Diagnostic cues generally are derived from the electrocardiogram (ECG) or 24-hour Holter monitor. It remains uncertain as to whether anti-arrhythmic therapy may regulate and limit the incidence of NSVT. Therefore, the diagnosis of NSVT is relevant principally in the context of a more general risk stratification of the patient, and similarly therapeutic strategies are aimed at optimizing long-term survivorship. A list of potential differential diagnoses is given (Table 1; Arrhythmia Alliance, 2010); these are identifiable by further history taking, examination, and investigation.

Non-sustained ventricular tachycardia (NSVT) is defined as a run of three or more consecutive ventricular beats at a rate of greater than or equal to 100 beats per minute, lasting for less than 30 seconds. In patients without structural heart disease, the incidence of NSVT is less common and can be seen in patients presenting with idiopathic ventricular ectopy or study populations from cardiac pacing trials. The appearance of NSVT during the acute setting of a cardiac event does not have the same prognostic significance as NSVT in patients with reduced left ventricular function, and it is thought that the latter accumulate a significantly greater pro-arrhythmic substrate.

3.1. Electrocardiogram (ECG) Findings

Non-required and unintended retrograde His bundle or right bundle branch activation in the intrinsic conduction represents the background of the intraventricular conduction abnormalities and permits to unmask structural cardiac diseases during tachycardia. Pathognomonic ECG features of idiopathic outflow-tract (OT) monomorphic ventricular tachycardias: lead I notching and Q waves and lead aVR monophasic R or QS with a short S-T segment are the hallmarks of an adrenergic-dependent Purkinje fascicular reentrant VT. PLC-related bundle branch block in both idiopathic fascicular tachycardias indicates a dilative cardiomyopathy. Wide QRS tachycardias fibrillating in respect to the PLC indicate a worse prognosis than those not fibrillating.

Discriminating between ventricular or supraventricular origin (focal or reentrant circuits). Evaluating the severity and intensity of the NSVT in relation to arrhythmic risk. The intact electrophysiological properties of the His-Purkinje system allow the QRS generated either by extra-stimulus or triggered complementary process during tachycardia to show a heterogeneous profile, and this explains the discrepancy between the seemingly narrow morphology of the initial beats and the markedly wider appearance of the terminal part of the successful propagating impulses (fusion). The fusion is a negative prognostic sign, and this finding must be considered also in post-infarction patients bearing the Pacifici's partial fascicular block.

The electrocardiogram (ECG) represents a cornerstone in the diagnosis and assessment of the arrhythmogenic substrates and triggers in patients suspected to have or already been diagnosed with non-sustained ventricular tachycardia (NSVT). Analysis of the ECG features originates from a cut point as prolonged QRS, reached during NSVT, and is potentially useful for two main aims:

3.2. Holter Monitoring

Holter monitoring provides a long-duration observation period that can identify these additional VT episodes compared with the more commonly used cardiac monitoring strategies. The NSTE-ACS subgroup of patients with ventricular tachycardia, including those with a self-limiting course, witnessed by an ECG in the setting of plaque ruptured type 1 myocardial infarction, are more likely to have reperfusion therapy as they present with increased urgency and worst underlying myocardial disease not tolerated the progressive ventricular electrical instability (class I, level A) as suggested by current guidelines. The 2020 stability-of-plan-strat-atrial-arrhythmias-ventricular-arrhythmias-algorithm defines NSVT as more than 8 beats at a rate more than 100 bpm and less than or equal to the rate for VT. The stability-of-plan-strat-atrial-arrhythmias-ventricular-arrhythmias-algorithm defines ventricular tachycardia (VT) as more than 30 s or sustained arrhythmia.

While many patients with non-sustained ventricular tachycardia (NSVT) may remain undiagnosed at initial presentment, these episodes of NSVT can be captured with several diagnostic tests over an extended monitoring period. One of the longest evaluations for capturing NSVT episodes is the Holter monitor. Rare arrhythmias such as NSVT can be underreported with shorter observational strategies. As a result, all patients with an ICD with a VTVF zone will have had manifest at least one episode of VT within a span of time to receive therapy. Similarly, once patients have had a second episode, this likely indicates that they are in a cycle of multiple arrhythmias that might be difficult to treat medically.

4. Treatment Options for NSVT

Medication is the typical first line treatment. The main objective of medical therapy is to control or prevent symptoms. Whether you have had recent events or not, there are a variety of antiarrhythmic medications which may be used per the discretion of the provider. As a general rule-of-thumb, the drug selected often depends on the antecedent cause of the patient's clinical syndrome. Providers will usually monitor your heart rhythm with serial ECGs/EKGs in the office at regular intervals to see if the antiarrhythmic therapy is suppressing the frequency of any symptoms or the seen heart rhythm event. Providers will also monitor a patient's clinical symptoms. It is likely that in patients with heart failure, beta blockers are used quite frequently, as they improve heart failure and also help suppress VT and VF episodes. If a patient has already been on a beta blocker, the dose can be increased or switched to a more potent agent like Sotalol. This approach appears to be effective at reducing the frequency of arrhythmia events. found that in a study of 233 patients, 86 (37%) patients had resolution of their inducible VT post beta blocker and Sotalol. Additionally, found that, in a study of 22 patients, 16 were treated with Sotalol monotherapy and 6 patients were treated with 3-drug therapy. In this group of 22 patients, 41.7% of the population had resolution of their inducible VT. While impressive, and anti-arrhythmics can effectively suppress VT burden, they are limited by side effects. Reversible anti-arrhythmics are best because they give the option of getting off the medication entirely should symptoms stop. If a catheter ablation is warranted, we increase the dose of antiarrhythmic to the maximum tolerated before the procedure. This significantly suppresses any arrhythmia within the first 3 months post-procedure.

Treatment for NSVT is geared towards either improving symptoms (feeling like the heart is racing or pounding) or treating potential eruption of fast VT. Conservative management consists of reassurance of safety in many cases given the good prognosis, and close monitoring for any worsening of symptoms or developing ventricular function decline. If there is concern for a potential more serious issue like a myocarditis that might have caused the NSVT or to evaluate for possible underlying scar in the heart, an MRI may be recommended. If there are concerning physical exam findings or signs of a more serious or significantly higher rate VT, a chest CT to exclude an active myocarditis can also be ordered. If a patient is found to be having a lot of NSVT or other ventricular arrhythmias on a monitor, a long loop monitor for 4 weeks may be used to get a "big picture" of all arrhythmias happening over that time frame, as trans-telephonic monitor (which only records for a short time and the data is "called in") likely does not give enough of a "snapshot" of what is going on.

4.1. Medications

Pharmacological management for non-sustained ventricular tachycardia (NSVT) should be handled in a multidisciplinary fashion between cardiologists and electrophysiologists (EP) to eliminate (if possible) the arrhythmia itself or treat the patient's clinical symptoms. A large variety of drugs are useful in both decreasing myocardial irritability and prolonging the refractory period, which significantly suppresses NSVT as well as the risk for ventricular fibrillation (VF). Refractory period (RP) is the time during regeneration of the action potential where the excitable cells of the heart cannot refire. Ideally, the RP is homogeneous throughout all the myocardial cells in the ventricle. RP can be prolonged by inhibiting open channels of sodium, potassium, and calcium or by inhibiting neurotransmitter and adrenoceptor activation. It is these receptor sites that different classes of medications target. The main classes of antiarrhythmics include β-blockers, calcium blockers, and class I, II, and IV medications. Anticoagulation treatment with warfarin should have a target INR between 2.0 and 3.0.

Medications as an approach to the treatment of non-sustained ventricular tachycardia (NSVT) are used with the goals of regulating the rhythm of the heart and treating related symptoms such as palpitations or lightheadedness. For most patients, especially if no definitive risk of future arrhythmias has been determined or if the frequency or duration of non-sustained ventricular tachycardia (NSVT) is low, medications are typically not used to directly suppress NSVT. Rather, medications are used to prevent sudden cardiac arrest by regulating the rhythm of the heart and preventing the development of potentially dangerous fast rhythms. Commonly used medications include β-blockers, which decrease the activity of the heart, slow the speed of conduction, and prolong repolarization. Antiarrhythmic medications, sometimes referred to as sodium or potassium channel blockers, suppress fast rhythms in the heart by acting on cells' "action potentials," which regulate the movement of charged ions essential for the heart to rhythmically beat.

4.2. Catheter Ablation

- Catheter ablation: procedural intervention with the aim of modifying cardiac tissue in a way that disrupts the current pathway of the arrhythmia or, in the case of focal arrhythmias, modifies substrates to prevent arrhythmogenesis. - Endpoints: may be immediate and include the loss of local injury potential, failure to reinduce ventricular tachycardia, non-inducibility of any ventricular tachycardia, or the inability to induce the clinical VT. Subsequent follow-up of recurrences could be useful, especially if there are alternate locations or foci generated. Requires preassessment with MRI and likely CAG to rule out unsuspected coronary artery or valvular disease. Often a multi-disciplinary input including external may also be useful. Careful patient counseling and optimization of medical therapy in the interim, as well as during follow-up.

In summary:

This will be achieved by targeting the culprit focus and encircling it with ablation lesions. The endpoint of ventricular tachycardia ablation will be non-inducibility in our patient. The procedure will be carried out under general anesthesia with para-magnetic defibrillation close to hand in view of the ventricular tachycardia. The three-dimensional mapping system will guide us to the focus. We will use steerable sheaths to construct the lesion overlay under the edges of the mitral valve and ivabradine dye will be delivered through the infusing catheter recommended to you by the surgeon. Pathways or ablation foci will be targeted until no inducible ventricular tachycardia is demonstrated. We will not target the Purkinje potential; in your conference with Dr. Aldo and Dr. William, they were not recruiting the Purkinje.

Catheter ablation is a procedure used to treat conditions of the heart. It uses a tool called a catheter to create pulses of energy that destroy the tissue causing the abnormal rhythm. Ablation is the main treatment option for non-sustained ventricular tachycardia. This is the procedure of choice in patients refractory or intolerant to antiarrhythmic therapy. It is often used in the case of ventricular tachycardia, a more advanced ventricular arrhythmia. Catheter ablation aims to modify cardiac tissue in a way that will either disrupt the current pathway of the arrhythmia or, in the case of focal arrhythmias, may modify substrates to prevent arrhythmogenesis. Given the nature of the illness in our elderly patient, we choose ablation of ventricular tachycardia in the left ventricle.

5. Prognosis and Life Expectancy

There are no definitive diagnostic criteria for non-sustained ventricular tachycardia (NSVT) nor treatment guidelines for individuals with NSVT in the absence of clinical disease. As a result, the estimated life expectancy for these individuals is largely driven by any other co-morbidities. Zipes and Johns, for instance, estimated that patients who had no underlying structural heart disease had a median survival with NSVT of 30 years compared with 21 years in controls without NSVT. However, Tasissa found that in the anoxic brain access visit, 39% of young, healthy patients with NSVT were concerned that they would live a shorter life because of their abnormal heartbeats, so this can be an opportunity to help relieve some of this anxiety by being understanding of their concerns. Given the benign prognosis of NSVT, many guidelines and expert opinions agree that the patient's primary care provider should assume the dominant role in their long-term care, and there is no need to schedule regular cardiac follow-up unless there are egregious risk factors presented.

One study found that while there was no difference in overall survival in patients with coronary artery disease and non-sustained ventricular tachycardia (NSVT) compared to those without NSVT over long-term follow-up, there was a nearly twofold increase in the risk of sudden cardiac death in patients with NSVT. In addition, five other studies established a disassociation between the occurrence of NSVT and an increased risk of sustained ventricular tachycardia (VT), sudden cardiac death, or complicated arrhythmic events.

5.1. Risk of Sudden Cardiac Death

The genesis of NSVT is related to the presence of reentrant circuits, the size of the area of slowed conduction, the presence of unidirectional conduction block within the circuit, and the short coupling interval which sometimes is able to reach the upstroke of the calcium channel-dependent premature beat before the increase in left ventricular segment volume. Reentry is favored by factors that affect impulse conduction in the circuit area, which may delay the return of the reentrant premature stimulus for the start of another cycle prior than expected. Fibrous intermyocardial connections make a unique anatomical and reentry microenvironment and potentially play a major role in this extremely vulnerable insulation heart scenario.

The frequency and extent of NSVT on ambulatory 24-hour Holter monitoring has been shown to be the most reproducible and reliable variable of all those proposed to be associated with increased risk of death from sudden arrhythmic causes. Non-sustained ventricular tachycardia represents a visible electrocardiographic marker of underlying myopathic injury and fibrosis. Fibrosis and necrosis trigger fractionation and slow conduction, which are the sine qua non of proarrhythmia. Sustained monomorphic VTs can cause not only syncope and sudden cardiac death but also be perceived by patients as palpitations and be associated with major decreases in quality of life.

5.2. Long-Term Outlook

In sum, NSVT treatment depends primarily on how NSVT came to light. If it is discovered simply as an incidental finding, it needs to be disadvantageous either for prognosis, symptoms, or potential therapies to warrant interest. The long-term outlook often establishes the prescription of activity restrictions and some medications, as more people with a benign outlook should be regarded as having restrictions or medications, by virtue of a greater burden of illness. We should expect that individuals undergoing long-term surveillance for NSVT would have more loads of ICD implants and limited activity prescriptions and be prioritized in the queue for more aggressive therapies, if more favorable illness-related details were available.

Most individuals discovered to have non-sustained ventricular tachycardia (NSVT) will have long-term stability with a benign outlook. This is even true for those with structural heart illness such as remote past myocardial infarction, mild valvular heart illness, or mild left ventricular dysfunction (LVEF 35-40%). Between 85% and 90% of individuals with NSVT have no symptoms referable to their arrhythmia. They do not have syncope nor are NSVT associated with psychological health (anxiety, depression) or impairments in quality-of-life scores. Or, at least, when NSVT surveillance is conducted in the aftermath of an initial hospitalization, the symptoms (such as cough, wheezing, flushing, and fainting) of patients with these symptoms are found to be far more helpful in anticipating future arrhythmic events than NSVT burden. One exception might be the younger age individuals with a family history of sudden death. Patients with repetitive, high-burden NSVT can be considered as a group that needs aggressive therapy for heart disease.